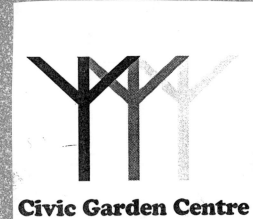

**Civic Garden Centre
Library**

Creating Fairy Garden Fragrances

LINDA GANNON

Illustrated by Dagmar Fehlau

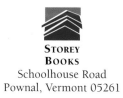

STOREY
BOOKS
Schoolhouse Road
Pownal, Vermont 05261

The mission of Storey Communications is to serve our customers by publishing practical information that encourages personal independence in harmony with the environment.

Dedication
For my children, Brittany, Kristin, Molly, and Austin,
who are no longer embarrassed to admit that their mother is the Faerie Queen!

Acknowledgments
I'd like to thank all the talented people at Storey who have helped make this book such a delightful adventure, especially my editors, Deborah Balmuth, who suggested that I write the book and gave me the creative freedom to do so, and Robin Catalano, who worked diligently to bring it all together; and all my supportive family and friends, especially my husband, Tom, who so wisely introduced me to the magic of the woods many years ago.

Edited by Deborah Balmuth and Robin Catalano
Cover design by Meredith Maker
Text design by E.K. Weymouth Design
Production assistance by Susan Bernier
Illustrations by Dagmar Fehlau
Line drawings on page 18 by Charles Joslin,
   page 19 by Brigita Fuhrmann

The information in this book is true and complete to the best of our knowledge. All recommendations are made without guarantee on the part of the author or Storey Books. The author and publisher disclaim any liability in connection with the use of this information. For additional information, please contact Storey Books, Schoolhouse Road, Pownal, Vermont 05261.

Storey Books are available for special premium and promotional uses and for customized editions. For further information, please call the Custom Publishing Department at 800-793-9396.

Printed in Hong Kong by C & C Offset Printing Co Ltd.
10 9 8 7 6 5 4 3 2 1

Library of Congress Cataloging-in-Publication Data

Gannon, Linda K., 1951–
    Creating Fairy Garden Fragrances / Linda K. Gannon
        p.   cm. — (The Spirit of aromatherapy)
        ISBN 1-58017-076-5 (alk. paper)
        1. Potpourris (Scented floral mixtures)
    2. Aromatherapy.   I. Title.   II. Series.
        TT899.4.G36   1998
        745.92—dc21   98-14495
                                                              CIP

Contents

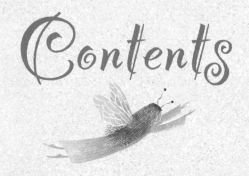

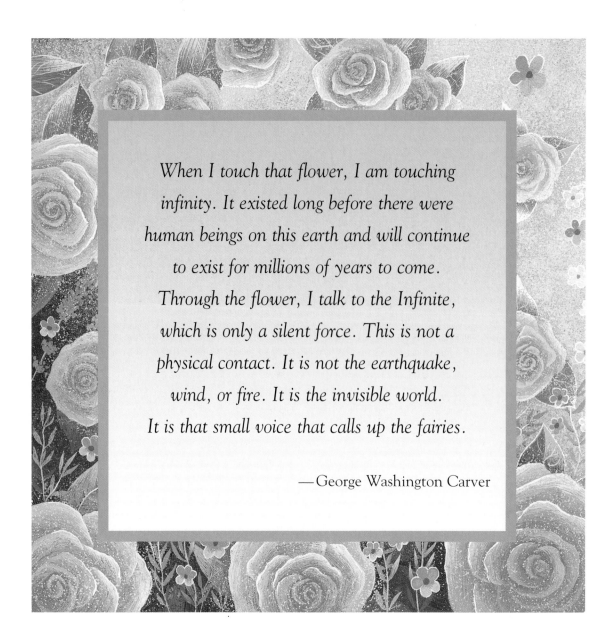

When I touch that flower, I am touching
infinity. It existed long before there were
human beings on this earth and will continue
to exist for millions of years to come.
Through the flower, I talk to the Infinite,
which is only a silent force. This is not a
physical contact. It is not the earthquake,
wind, or fire. It is the invisible world.
It is that small voice that calls up the fairies.

—George Washington Carver

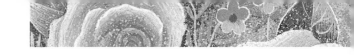

The Realm of Fairies

Fairies and flowers and magic are interwoven in a rich and ancient tapestry. I've known this since the earliest days of my life, when my favorite nature books were tales of fantasy in which fairies danced with dragonflies, slept beneath toadstools, and granted wishes in enchanted gardens. The flowers were lush with color and fragrance; birds sang, honeybees hummed, and dew collected to form moonpools in the tightly curled leaves of the captivating plants.

I was in awe of this magic kingdom, and would often let my imagination transport me into the realm of my books. It was here in the mystical forests that I first frolicked with the fairies among the primroses and wild thyme in midsummer joy.

My favorite sojourn into the garden took place one sultry summer night. A nearly full moon shone silver wisps upon the mist, and elfin silhouettes stood stark against the luminous sky. There was an absolute spellbound stillness, the garden became a sanctuary, and I stood rooted to the mossy ground, absorbing memories of the long-forgotten magic of the earth — secrets that lie within the enchanted foxglove and sacred vervain.

It was at that moment that I began to feel a powerful presence of life in another time and another place — a connection to an invisible realm where nature, divinity, underworld, and human world became one.

Fairy Lore

My storybooks were soon replaced with folklore journals, and I discovered ancient stories about those who inhabited this supernatural world.

The wee folk of this kingdom were known by various names, depending upon which part of the world you were from, and of which type of spirit you spoke. The Irish fairies were known as *sidhe*, the good people, or good neighbors. Ancient Celtic people who lived close to the earth considered their fairies to be both companions and powerful forces in their lives. Brownies and elves were the working fairies of English medieval origin, and would often adopt a household and look after it. *Siths*, also known as pixies, played that role for the Scots. Mannikins had a strong connection to trees and wildflowers, and may have been the fairies young Will Shakespeare wrote of so poetically.

Greek undines (usually female in form) and Scottish kelpies (who often took the form of horses) belonged to the water. Sylphs were the nature spirits of Greece whose elements were wind, clouds, and storms. *Devas,* or the "shining ones," were nature spirits from Persia who were believed to appear as bright spheres of light.

Fauns, satyrs, dryads, and other mythical beasts of Greece were the mischievious sort who played their pranks during the night; leprechauns were the Irish practical jokers. Native Americans believed every living thing had a spirit that revealed itself in animal form. These animal "fairies" aided the tribespeople's understanding of the cycles of life, death, and rebirth.

In folklore records, fairies are nearly always credited with having a mysterious habitation underground and, in the case of kelpies and watersprites, underwater. There are also legends of fairies inhabiting trees, of which they shared a strong affection for rowan and elder (under which True Thomas, in Edmund Spenser's famous poem, encountered the Faerie Queene).

The traditional fairy circle, in which you must stand if you wish to experience magic, consists of oak, ash, and hawthorn.

Fairy Tales

In 1646, a young English woman by the name of Anne Jefferies claimed she was surrounded by six tiny green men as she sat knitting beneath an elder tree at the entrance to her arbor. The most handsome of the bunch jumped into her palm, then onto her bosom, and began kissing her neck. Entranced, she felt herself transported through the air and then plunked into a wonderous garden filled with wee people. A short while later, she awoke in her arbor, surrounded by worried friends.

Anne's tale arose suspicion of falsehood and she was soon imprisoned. After her release, she never spoke of the episode again.

In a similar story in the English Folklore Record of 1878, there was a report of the fashionable Victorian baths being patronized by fairies. One lovely summer morning when William Butterfield went to unlock the doors to the spa, they stuck as though being held on the other side. With a great heave, William pushed the doors open, and there in the silvery light were dozens of tiny green men, all dripping wet! William called out to them, but, frightened, they scattered in all directions. Within seconds the fairies were gone, and the pool was tranquil. Not a trace remained of their mysterious visit.

There is also a legend from Germany about an elf that inhabited the Hubichenstein Hills. One day, the wife of a poor, sick miner went out to gather some beautiful fir cones, in hopes of trading them for money. In the forest she met a little man with a long white beard, who told her where the best cones could be found. At the place he spoke of, she was deluged with cones; terrified, she ran away. When she later looked at the cones that had fallen into her basket, she found they had turned to pure silver.

She returned to the woods the next day, where the little man — Gubich, King of the Dwarves — gave her some herbs that later restored her husband to health. The newly wealthy miner preserved one of his silver cones. It is said that the cone can be found in the Grund (now the Museum of Mineralogy) to this day.

Cottingley, England, is the setting for the famous story of Elsie Wright and Frances Griffiths, who would often talk of playing with prism-winged pixies in the wood behind their home. So one day in 1917, Elsie's father gave her his camera and told the girls to photograph the fairies. Upon developing the plate, he was astonished to see Frances with a whole flock of fairies dancing around her.

News of the photos spread to a man named Edward Gardner, who believed in nature spirits on earth, which he called "elementals." He took quite an interest in the girls' story and, with the help of his friend Sir Arthur Conan Doyle (of Sherlock Holmes fame), had the photos published in *Strand* magazine.

Predictably, the photos caused a stir among the public; the skeptical believed they somehow had been enhanced in the photography studio. Doyle and Gardner, however, were among those completely convinced that the fairies were real, and both later wrote books to elaborate on the girls' encounters. These books were published by the Theosophical Society of England in 1945.

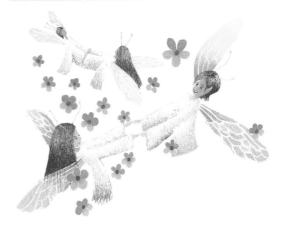

Fairy Friends

Among Sir Arthur Conan Doyle's musings were these words that prophesied about the incredible impact the reality of fairies would have in our world. He wrote:

"These little folk who appear to be our neighbors, with only some small difference of vibration to separate us, will become familiar. The thought of them, even when unseen, will add charm to every brook and valley and give romantic interest to every country walk."

The Findhorn Gardens

Probably the most recent and well-documented communication with the supernatural world is the story of the Findhorn Gardens. In 1962 Peter and Eileen Caddy, a couple of young clairvoyants, were "guided" to Findhorn Caravan Park, Morayshire, in the bleak north of Scotland, to a site little more than a rubbish heap. Claiming that they had received instructions from the *devas*, the Caddys planted a garden on this barren land.

And then astonishing things happened: cabbages tipped the scales at 40 pounds; delphiniums growing in pure sand grew to a height of 8 feet; and roses commonly bloomed amid snow and ice.

John Aubrey, in his book Miscellanies, *writes of a fairy encounter:*

> "Anno 1670, not far from Cirencester, was an apparition; being demanded whether a good spirit or bad? returned no answer, but disappeared with a curious perfume and most melodious twang. Mr W. Lilly believes it was a fairy."

The Fairy Corner

There were mysteries of other kinds at Findhorn as well. Sheds appeared precisely when needed, and warnings were sounded just on the brink of disaster. One morning some paths were being rid of gorse when suddenly, the Greek god Pan appeared with a message. The nature spirits were angry at the humans for destroying their homes, and were preparing to flee the garden. Pan taught the gardeners how important it was for them to work in communion with the spirits of the earth. It was vital, he said, to leave a small area of the garden wild and undisturbed so the fairies would have a private place in which to dwell.

I agree, as many gardeners do, that the legendary Pan knew of what he spoke: that leaving a patch of earth untilled, unplanted, and untouched will allow the magical flowers to grow as they please, and insects, wildlife, and the fairies will claim it as their home. So many beautiful things that are out of place or will not flourish in the sophistication of a formal bed will thrive here to charm us with their blossoms, as well as their lore.

Flowers of the Fairies

Bluebells, cowslips, forget-me-nots, fox-glove, pansies, periwinkle, primroses, ragwort, vervain, wood sorrel, and, of course, toadstools are all considered to be fairy flowers, having legendary associations with the wee folk of nature.

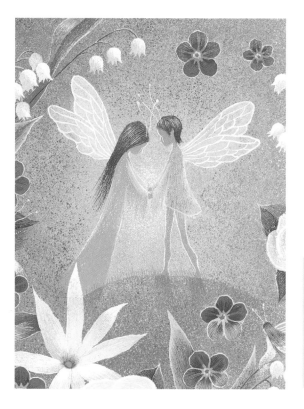

Shakespeare tells us also of oxlips, roses, violets, woodbine (honeysuckle), and eglantine, the lovely name for sweetbrier.

Folklore, too, describes flowers that were included in the "fairy garland." Cuckooflowers, ground flax, harebells, mallow, and stitchwort are some of the lesser-known wildlings that might also be part of this magical garden. These, along with hosts of others, will fill a tiny wood or glade you've chosen as the fairy corner and bring joy throughout the seasons.

And if you visit this sacred spot and a tiny green bug alights on your shoulder, it just might be that diminutive elf we've talked about, come from another realm to whisper words of wisdom — a prayer for nonbelievers: Learn to work in harmony with our blessed planet, and it will sustain and nourish us.

In the Victorian botanical "language," the gift of flowers takes on a specific meaning:

Forget-me-not — *Loving remembrance and fidelity*
Lavender — *Devotion*
Lily-of-the-valley — *Purity*
Roses — *Love and desire*

Faerie Flora

Within the magical blends that follow, you will find many uses for these fairy flowers. Some you will want to grow yourself, but many can be uncovered along roadsides and in woodlands. Because they are not critical ingredients to the blends, but rather magical additives, do not despair if you are unable to locate them. Traditional flowers and herbs will make up the bulk of the blends.

Balsam fir

(*Abies balsamea*). The scent from balsam needles is reminiscent of the heady, crisp aroma of a forest. Its inexpensive essential oil provides a wonderful way to bring the outdoors in!

Bay

(*Laurus nobilis*). An evergreen tree native to the Mediterranean region, bay has beautiful pale green leaves that have a delicious, spicy aroma whether fresh or dried. The essential oil is crisp and sharp.

Bergamot

(*Citrus aurantium* subsp. *bergamia*). This small fruit, which resembles a lemon, grows chiefly in West India. Its essential oil is expressed from the peel and yields a wonderfully refreshing, citrusy fragrance.

Bergamot mint

(*Mentha × piperita* var. *citrata*). The leaves of this scarlet spring flower produce a crisp, citrusy aroma loved by insects and hummingbirds. No essential oil is available.

Calendula

(*Calendula officinalis*). The bright yellow-orange flowers keep their vivid color when dried and retain a faint aroma. Calendula oil is actually an infused oil.

Cardamom

(*Elettaria cardamomum*). Cardamom is the second most expensive spice in common world trade; only saffron is costlier. Its dried seeds and essential oil produce a most luxuriant, sweetly intoxicating scent.

Cedar

(*Cedrus atlantica*). In ancient Lebanon, cedar was highly prized for its rich scent, so much so that few trees now remain. The essential oil and dried needles have a deep, woodsy aroma.

Cinnamon

(*Cinnamomum cassia*). The delicately spicy, sweet aroma from the dried inner bark of the Chinese cinnamon tree, cassia (which is actually an inferior spice), is also the fragrance of the essential oil.

Clove

(*Syzygium aromaticum*). The unopened red buds produce the ultimate spicy essential oil of this, one of the most aromatic culinary spices.

Cuckooflower

(*Cardamine pratensis*). A member of the cress family, the wild cuckooflower makes a silver splash in a wet corner of the yard where little else will grow. No essential oil is available.

Deer's-tongue

(*Frasera speciosa*). The delicious, vanilla-like, sensual fragrance comes from the twisty dried leaves. No essential oil is available.

Forget-me-not

(*Myosotis scorpioides* var. *semperflorens*). Dainty true blue flowers with yellow eyes, forget-me-nots make a beautiful woodland ground cover. Many fairy legends are associated with these charmers, most dealing with remembrance. No essential oil is available.

Foxglove

(*Digitalis* × *mertonensis*). The tall spires of pastel, bell-shaped foxglove make it a coveted garden wildflower. It is probably the most legendary of fairy flowers. No essential oil is available.

Honeysuckle

(*Lonicera caprifolium*). The scent of this pretty twining vine is considered an aphrodisiac. The essential oil is luxuriantly sweet and soothing.

Hyacinth

(*Hyacinthus orientalis*). An early-spring bloomer, its tiny blossoms produce an incredibly lovely scent. No true essential oil is available, but imitations are easily made from blends.

Jasmine

(*Jasminum grandiflorum*). This is a beautiful white, night-flowering plant from China. It is exquisitely aromatic — and exquisitely expensive. The true essential oil is worth the splurge.

Juniper

(*Juniperus communis*). Juniper was burned for the gods and goddesses in ancient Babylon, and is still widely used in incense formulas. The crushed, dried berries and essential oil have a pungent, pinelike aroma.

Lavender

(*Lavandula angustifolia* subsp. *angustifolia*). The fresh purple flowers, dried flowers, and essential oil all have a fresh, clean, soothing aroma. One of the most versatile scents.

Lemon verbena

(*Aloysia triphylla*). Originally from Chile, lemon verbena has a heavenly lemon scent found in the pale green leaves. The essential oil is expensive, but well worth the cost.

Lily-of-the-valley

(*Convallaria majalis*). The dainty, bell-shaped spring flowers emit a lightly sweet, pleasant scent. No essential oil is available.

Neroli

(*Citrus aurantium*). Also known as orange flower, neroli has a heady, rich essence that is distilled from flowers of the bitter orange tree. The essential oil is incredibly expensive, but worth every penny.

Oakmoss

(*Evernia prunastri*). A lichen that grows on oak trees, it has a gray-green color that is beautiful in woodsy blends. The essential oil smells of seaside plants and damp woods.

Pansy

(*Viola × wittrockiana*). The "little flower with a face" comes in a variety of vivid colors and with a heritage of fairy folklore. No essential oil is available.

Patchouli

(*Pogostemon cablin*). A popular, evocative scent in the psychedelic '60s, patchouli's essential oil and dried leaves have a deep, rich, earthy sweetness.

Periwinkle

(*Vinca minor*). The familiar woodland ground cover bears blue flowers in spring, and was once thought to possess magical powers. No essential oil is available.

Pine

(*Pinus sylvestris*). The clean, exhilarating pine-forest fragrance is captured in the dried needles, as well as in the essential oil.

Primrose

(*Oenothera biennis*). The delicate, pale pink blossoms open as the sun is setting on this edible wildflower, often called the fairy flower. No essential oil is available.

Queen-Anne's-lace

(*Daucus carota*). Tiny white clusters form a lacy flower head on this beautiful "weed." The fragrance is strong; its taste is bitter. No essential oil is available.

Rose

(*Rosa damascena; R. centifolia*). The blossoms of this "queen of flowers" produce the quintessential sweet fragrance. Traditionally distilled to produce essential oil (attar), rose essence is also extracted through a solvent (absolute).

Sandalwood

(*Santalum album*). Grown commercially in India, sandalwood has an incredible warm, woodsy, mysterious scent. The wood, root, and essential oil have long been used for incense.

Sassafras

(*Sassafras albidum*). This plant is native to the eastern United States. The essential oil produced from the root bark is spicy and stimulating.

Spearmint

(*Mentha spicata*). The minty fresh flowers, dried leaves, and essential oil are used in potpourri for their mild stimulating effect.

Sweet pea

(Lathyrus odoratus). With pastel blossoms in nearly every color except yellow, the dainty sweet pea is exquisitely sweet. No essential oil is available.

Sweet woodruff

(Galium odoratum). The beautiful dark green dried leaves emit a warm, vanilla-like aroma. No essential oil is available.

Thyme

(Thymus vulgaris). This pungent-scented herb grows as a ground cover. It has lovely lavender blossoms, in which it is said fairies hide their babies for safekeeping! The essential oil has an antiseptic aroma and is used medicinally.

Toadstool

(Marasmius oreades). There are many folk tales linking the rapid-growing, luminous, often poisonous toadstools with fairies. Definitely no essential oil is available!

Tonka

(Dipteryx odorata). Tonka's dried brown beans emit a wonderfully rich, vanilla fragrance. Be careful: They are toxic, so do not ingest. No essential oil is available.

Tuberose

(Polianthes tuberosa). Native to Mexico, this plant produces intensely fragrant, waxy white flower spikes that are most aromatic at night. The essential oil is made by enfleurage, a complex and expensive procedure, so it is difficult to find.

Vanilla

(Vanilla planifolia). An orchid indigenous to Central America, this plant produces a pod that, once dried and cured, creates vanillin. Natural vanilla oil is hard to come by, so we use the delicious, sweet-smelling beans.

Vervain

(Verbena hastata). Legend holds that this inconspicuous herb was sacred to fairies and priests, for it drove away evil spirits. It also had many medicinal uses. No essential oil is available.

Vetiver

(Vetiveria zizanioides). The dried ground rootstock of this tall grass produces a rich, woodsy, and uplifting essential oil.

Wood sorrel

(Oxalis acetosella). Believed to be the true shamrock of the ancient Druids, this plant has delicate white blossoms and thrives in the fairy woodlands. No essential oil is available.

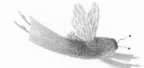

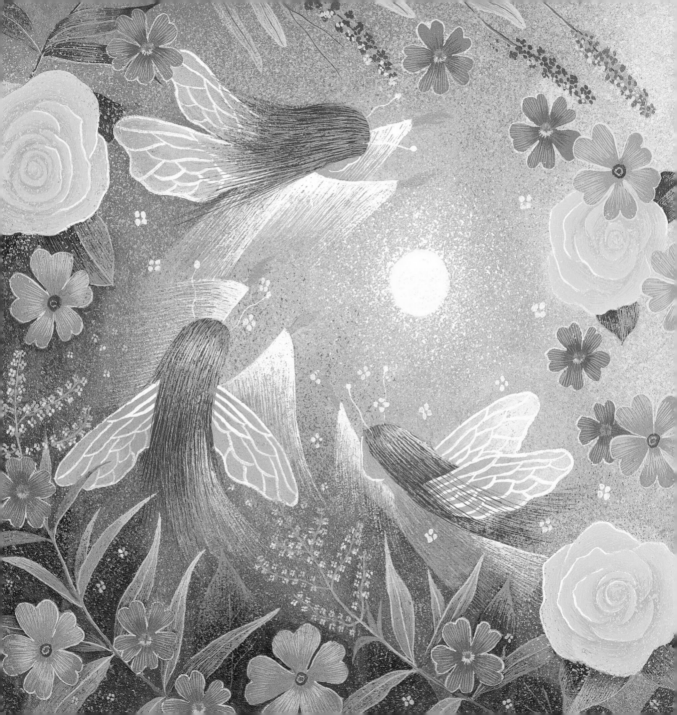

Essential Oils

Essential oils intensify or complement the fragrance of your blends. True essential oils are, in actuality, concentrated plant energies. Just as in animals nerves transmit fine impulses, and glands secrete minute amounts of active substances in an involuntary process, so, too, does the essential oil perform these roles in plant life. Essential oils are obtained from blossoms, leaves, stems, and rootstock by steam distillation, enfleurage, extraction, and expression. These are all very costly and potentially dangerous procedures; it is best to leave them to the professionals.

Many distributors sell synthetic oils and essences. These are man-made approximations of a plant's aroma, and have nothing to do with living plant material. True essential oils are born of living plants, nourished by soil, sun, and rain; they vibrate with the subtle energy of our earth. There is an aesthetic quality to them that synthetic oils can never attain.

Genuine essential oils are usually sold in milliliter amounts, and vary in cost from inexpensive — bergamot, lemon, pine — to very expensive — jasmine, neroli, rose. Though many true essential oils are initially expensive to obtain, they are used in such tiny amounts that their overall price is actually minimal.

Once you have purchased your essential oils, treat them as something precious. Keep them out of direct sunlight, away from direct heat, firmly capped, and in a cool, dry place. If treated with care, the oils can remain viable for several years.

Often, you can find premixed essential oil combinations from botanical and fragrance companies. These are wonderful and will save you the experimentation stage of finding compatible scents if the company is reputable.

Handling Essential Oils

Remember, essential oils are highly concentrated forms of the plant from which they are extracted, and you could be susceptible to allergic reactions; use all new oils with caution. It is always best to protect your skin from direct contact with the oils, and do not ingest!

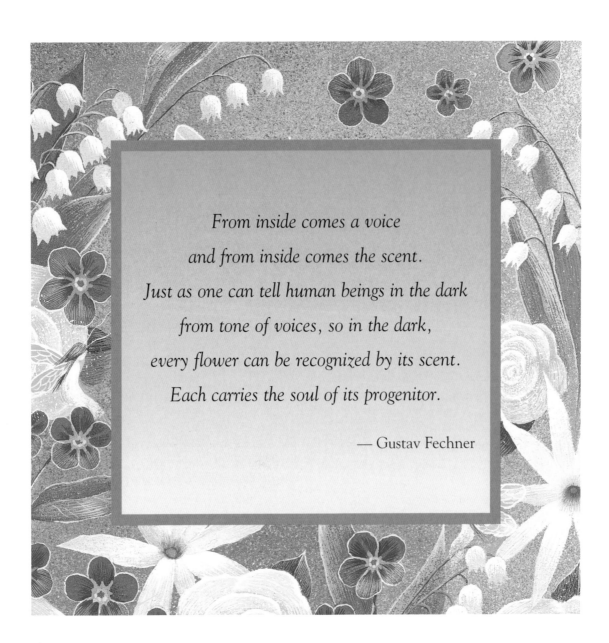

From inside comes a voice
and from inside comes the scent.
Just as one can tell human beings in the dark
from tone of voices, so in the dark,
every flower can be recognized by its scent.
Each carries the soul of its progenitor.

— Gustav Fechner

Celebrating the Seasons with Fairy Fragrance

The word *potpourri* means "a mixture of many ingredients." We use the term today to refer to a mixture of flowers with herbal greenery — sometimes this also includes berries, cones, fruit, pods, and spices — that are blended to gently and subtly perfume the air. I imagine that potpourri has been made for almost as long as flowers have been cultivated, for it is a way of preserving a flower's fragrance long after its blooming life has ended. Often, we create scents to stimulate a memory or send us off into fantastic dreams.

The changing seasons of our earth provide fertile ground for evocative aromas. Spring brings the promise of the sweet perfume of lilacs and apple blossoms. The warm, sultry fragrances of narcissus, roses, and freshly mown grass send sensual messages of summer days. The smell of wet maple leaves conjures memories of autumn. And who can inhale the fresh aroma of balsam and not picture the wonders of winter?

Gathering the Flowers and Herbs

Gather flowers and herbs for drying on clear dry days, after the dew has evaporated. Always pick the blossoms that have *just* reached their peak, when their essential oils and colors are at their fullest and brightest.

Begin to harvest whatever you can in spring, such as daffodils, freesia, hyacinths, lilacs, lilies-of-the-valley, narcissus, peonies, primroses, violets, and wild geraniums. Continue into summer with black-eyed Susans, carnations, coneflowers, delphiniums, forget-me-nots, heliotrope, honeysuckle, jasmine, lavender, mint, pansies, Queen-Anne's-lace, rosemary, roses, scented geraniums, and sweet peas. Autumn will bring berries, colored leaves, cones, mosses, pods, and vines. And in winter you'll find arborvitae, balsam, boxwood, cedar, juniper, and other fresh greens to use in festive holiday blends.

Drying the Flowers and Herbs

You can dry the flowers whole or spread the petals on screens in a warm, dry, dark room. It may be necessary to turn the flowers every so often until they are dry. In just a few days, the blossoms will be crisp to the touch and ready to store in jars, where they should be kept until it is time to use them in your blends.

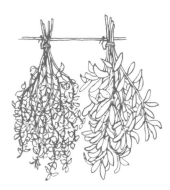

Greens and grasses can be cut and dried the same way, or you can tie them in small bunches to hang upside down in a warm, dry, dark place. This works well if space is a problem; plant material will just take a little longer to dry.

I like to add dried fruit to my autumn and winter potpourris. They provide the fruity fragrance, color, and texture that is so appropriate to the waning seasons of the year. Dry lemons, limes, oranges, and pomegranates whole by putting them somewhere warm and dry. It will take a couple of months for these to dry completely, so put them in a closet in August or September and forget about them until October, when you're ready to mix your harvest blend. You can also slice apples, lemons, limes, or oranges and dry them in a couple of days in an electric food dehydrator. Or lay them on screens for a week or so in that same warm, dry, dark room with your flowers.

Once you have accumulated the dried bounty, you are ready to begin designing your potpourri.

> *The drier the room, the quicker the flowers and fruits will dry, and the more color and fragrance your final product will retain.*

Creating the Enchanted Mixtures

The secret to creating a luscious mixture is to blend a harmonious perfume from several different aromas. So begin the process of creating blends by choosing flowers and herbs with scents that you like.

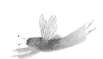

1. Select and Mix the Flowers and Herbs

Mix flowers and herbs that are pleasing to your olfactory sense, but keep color in mind as well. When you are satisfied with your plant blend, you are ready to add the essential oils.

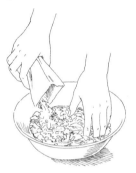

2. Combine Essential Oils with a Fixative

I like to add my oils to a fixative (a fragrance preservative) before adding them to the flower mixture; it not only holds the volatile oils, but also distributes them evenly over the petals, allowing the aromas to mingle and mellow.

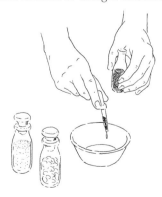

Recommended Fixatives

Calamus root (from sweet flag) adds a spicy quality.

Frankincense and **myrrh** (tree resins) have sharp balsam scents that work well with woodsy blends.

Ground cinnamon or **cloves** are readily available and will bring a gorgeous rich scent to the mixture.

Gum benzoin (a resinous gum) is very aromatic and complements floral scents.

Oakmoss is a lichen that yields a resin that acts as a preservative; especially effective with fruity blends.

Orrisroot (the rootstock of the iris) has a wonderful violet-like scent, but is known to be toxic to many people.

Storax, like other balsams, adds a "low note" to the potpourri.

Tonka beans have a very rich, vanilla-like fragrance.

In a large glass jar or earthenware crock, add your base oil — the oil that will carry the "theme" of your blend — to the fixative, normally 15 to 20 drops, then other oils 1 drop at a time until you have exactly the scent you desire. I usually use about 30 to 35 drops of oil total for ¼ cup of fixative. This is enough to generously perfume 6 cups of mixture. Cover securely, shake gently to mix, and let the oils and fixative blend 2 to 3 days before using. If blended correctly, the scent will last long after the flowers in the mixture have faded.

3. Put It All Together with Textured Elements

Pour the flowers and herbs into the container with your essential oils/fixative mixture. Now it's time to add any dried berries, fruits, nuts, pods, pinecones, woods, and vines that will give your potpourri texture, as well as charm. Like supporting notes in a symphony, these magical additions embellish the basic character of the blend's bouquet.

Once you are satisfied that your mixture is irresistible, cover your crock or jar, gently invert several times to mix, then allow it to "cure" for about four weeks. You will soon have a magical garden still abloom when all others are on the wane.

Use the same, simple directions for each blend.

Finishing Touches

These are fairy mixtures, so toss in anything of whimsy and everything that glitters! Always add the finishing touches after you have combined your floral mixture with the essential oils, fixative, and textured elements.

I will often "gild" (spray gently with gold paint) pinecones, fruits, and winter greens to give the blend a magical glow.

A few pressed and gilded flowers are a delightful and dazzling addition; pressed butterflies and dragonflies are especially enchanted, if you can find them!

CHOOSING THE RIGHT FRAGRANCE MIX

FLOWERS AND HERBS

Sweet/Floral
carnation
freesia
gardenia
heliotrope
honeysuckle
hyacinth
jasmine
lilac
lily-of-the-valley
magnolia
narcissus
rose
scented geranium
sweet pea
tuberose
violet

Fruity
apple blossom
lemon balm
lemon flower
lemon verbena leaf
lime blossom
orange blossom
scented geranium
   blossom and leaf

Green/Herbal
bee balm
chamomile
clary sage
lavender
orange mint
peppermint
rosemary
sage
spearmint
sweet marjoram
sweet woodruff
thyme

Woodsy/Spicy
cedar
cinnamon
deer's-tongue
ginger
patchouli
sandalwood
tonka
vanilla
vetiver

ESSENTIAL OILS

Sweet/Floral
frangipani
gardenia
honeysuckle
hyacinth
jasmine
rose
tuberose
violet
ylang-ylang

Fruity
bergamot
cardamom
citronella
lemon
lemon balm
lemongrass
lemon verbena
lime
mandarin orange
neroli
petitgrain
tangerine

Green/Herbal
basil
balsam fir
clary sage

eucalyptus
lavender
marjoram
peppermint
Peru balsam
rosemary
sage
spearmint
sweet woodruff

Woodsy/Spicy
bay
birch
calamus root
cedar
cinnamon
clove
cypress
eucalyptus
frankincense
ginger
juniper berry
myrrh
nutmeg
patchouli
rosemary
rosewood
sandalwood
vetiver

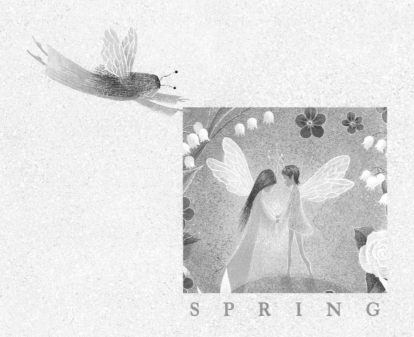

SPRING

Spring Fragrances

The circular journey of nature begins with the
possibilities and promises of springtime, exuberant
with new life — fragrant, fresh, and tender.
The sherbet hues of daffodils, lavender, lilacs,
lilies-of-the-valley, primroses, violets, and the prettiest
pale green grasses welcome this sparkling new year.
Birds, bugs, and the spring peepers in love
will serenade us in celebration!

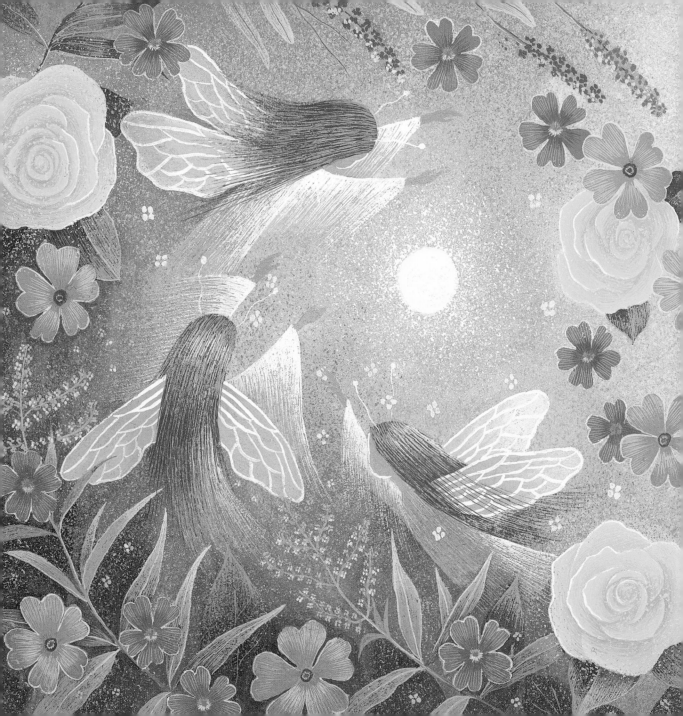

Dance of the Morning Nymphs

Softly, like a baby's breath, the dawn begins to whisper, promising

another perfect day. The tender flowers unfold their petals

to bask in the sunshine. Crickets sing, dragonflies dance, dew still

clings to the lush, fragrant flowers. The morning fairies

stir as we eavesdrop on the murmurings of the earth beginning

its sweet celebration of awakening and renewal . . .

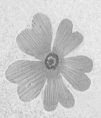

This blend is innocently exuberant — a combination of heady rose, tangy lemon, and luscious green cardamom, splashed with a hint of vivacious bergamot mint. Shades of pale greens, pure yellows, and lavender make it a perfect gift for all new beginnings and spring celebrations.

Dance of the Morning Nymphs

Dried Flowers and Herbs

    2 cups yellow rosebuds
    2 cups lemon verbena leaves
    1 cup lavender flowers
    ½ cup bergamot mint leaves

Essential Oils

    20 drops lemon verbena oil
    10 drops rose oil
    5 drops lavender oil

Fixative

    ¼ cup ground calamus root

Textured Elements

    ¼ cup green cardamom pods

Finishing Touches

    ½ cup primrose blossoms
    ½ cup wood sorrel blossoms
    ¼ cup gold star confetti

Package the blend in a small cut-crystal bowl tied up with opulent lemon yellow or pale green French ribbon. Glorious!

Evening primrose

The beautifully symmetrical "stars" of the edible pink primrose bloom early in the spring. They are among the first "fairy flowers" to salute the new season.

As its name suggests, the primrose blooms as the sun is setting, and by the next morning its delicate petals are wilted and spent. Some 19th-century botanists believed that the flowers of the evening primrose were phosphorescent. Others believed they stored sunlight during the day, and that accounted for their unusual visibility at night.

Also called the Evening Star, primrose inspired one poet to write:

> *"You Evening Primroses, when day*
> *has fled,*
> *Open your pallid flowers, by dew and*
> *moonlight fed."*

Wood sorrel

The delicate blush of white petals — veined red or deep pink as a guide for insects — bloom atop beautiful, pale green, heart-shaped leaves that herbalists once used to treat heart conditions. Wood sorrel, which thrives in the woodlands, blooms during the Easter season, and thus it has become a symbol for rebirth. Wood sorrel is believed to be the true shamrock, an ancient Druidic symbol that St. Patrick employed to explain the Trinity when he arrived to spread Christianity in Ireland in 432.

Because its leaves close up at night, it has also been called sleeping beauty. The Welsh call the plant fairy bells, believing its bell-shaped blossoms summoned elves to moonlight revelry.

The Wedding of
Titania and ☾Oberon

Fairy Queen Titania and King Oberon seal their troth
atop a small, mossy garden knoll encircled by lush white
wedding roses and vines of seductive jasmine in full bloom,
with the rich, gorgeous scent heavy on the breeze . . .
The elves in attendance sway gently on the enticing lemon
verbena, holding tight to their tiny bouquets of
lilies-of-the-valley and fresh forget-me-nots.
The electricity of love and magic fills the hillside!

This blend is elegant yet romantic in buttercream
flower buds, silvery greens, and a hint of azure. It is
harmoniously sweet and sensual.

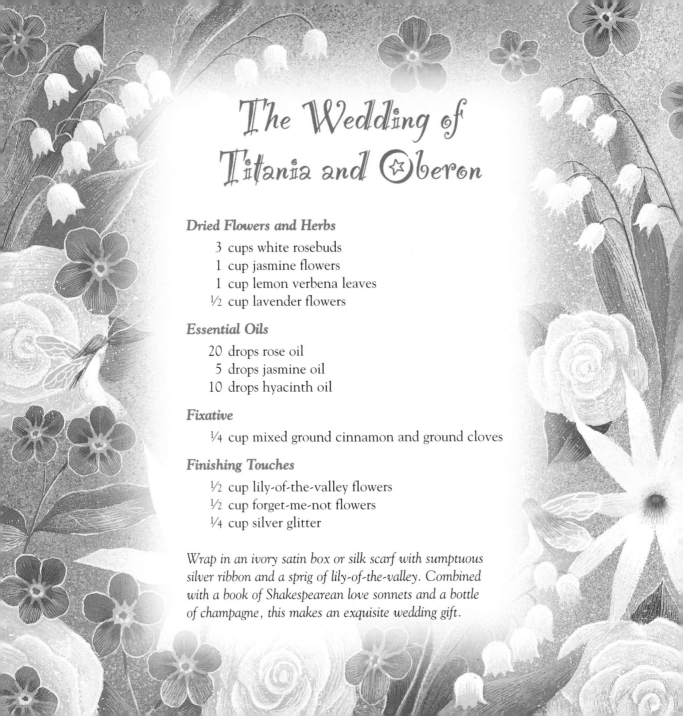

The Wedding of Titania and Oberon

Dried Flowers and Herbs

    3 cups white rosebuds
    1 cup jasmine flowers
    1 cup lemon verbena leaves
    ½ cup lavender flowers

Essential Oils

    20 drops rose oil
     5 drops jasmine oil
    10 drops hyacinth oil

Fixative

    ¼ cup mixed ground cinnamon and ground cloves

Finishing Touches

    ½ cup lily-of-the-valley flowers
    ½ cup forget-me-not flowers
    ¼ cup silver glitter

Wrap in an ivory satin box or silk scarf with sumptuous silver ribbon and a sprig of lily-of-the-valley. Combined with a book of Shakespearean love sonnets and a bottle of champagne, this makes an exquisite wedding gift.

Lily-of-the-valley

Tiny white, fragrant bells grow on this sweet spring-blooming wildflower. Much Christian symbolism surrounds its creation. One medieval legend tells of St. Leonard, who lived in the forest. The dragon Temptation, who lived nearby, burned down St. Leonard's hut. A fierce battle ensued, and wherever St. Leonard's blood fell, a beautiful lily-of-the-valley appeared.

Considered a symbol of purity, humility, and sweetness, the lily-of-the-valley is also called ladder to heaven, Jacob's tears, and Mary's tears (some believed that when Mary cried at the cross, the tears turned to lily-of-the-valley blossoms).

Forget-me-not

One of the few pure blue flowers that exist in nature, the tiny ground-covering forget-me-not is truly enchanting.

In almost every culture there is a tale connected with the forget-me-not. In one widely told story, a knight and his lover were walking along a stream when he saw some beautiful blue flowers growing on the other side. He jumped into the water, armor and all, and managed to grab some of the flowers and toss them to his sweetheart before going under. His final words: "Forget me not."

The forget-me-not is associated today with loving remembrance, friendship, and fidelity.

In Christian legend, God named all the plants during the six days of creation, but the little blue flower with the yellow eye could not remember her name. Finally, God whispered, "Forget me not, that is your name!"

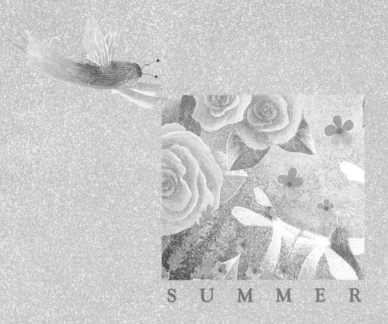

SUMMER

Summer Fragrances

In rushes summer, bursting with color and fragrance.

Each day awakens us to immense surprises

and mysteries, lest we forget we live

in a wondrous universe!

Delphiniums, forget-me-nots, honeysuckle,

hyacinths, jasmine, narcissus, pansies, roses,

and sweet peas scent the sultry days

and nights with their heady perfume.

Pan's Song

Imagine the alluring beauty of a cottage rose garden

growing in wild abundance, miniature fairies hovering over

each budding blossom, their sweetness the sum of warm

summer days and careful tending. The moss-covered walls

are beginning to crumble from the weight of the

tangled vines. Here and there among hidden patches of thyme

lie tiny footprints embedded among the blossoms.

Pan's Song is sensual and sweet with rose, an
alluring hint of lemon, and subtle thyme tossed
in. It is gorgeous in shades of pink with a wee
touch of lavender.

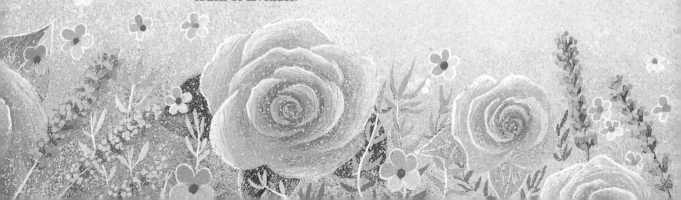

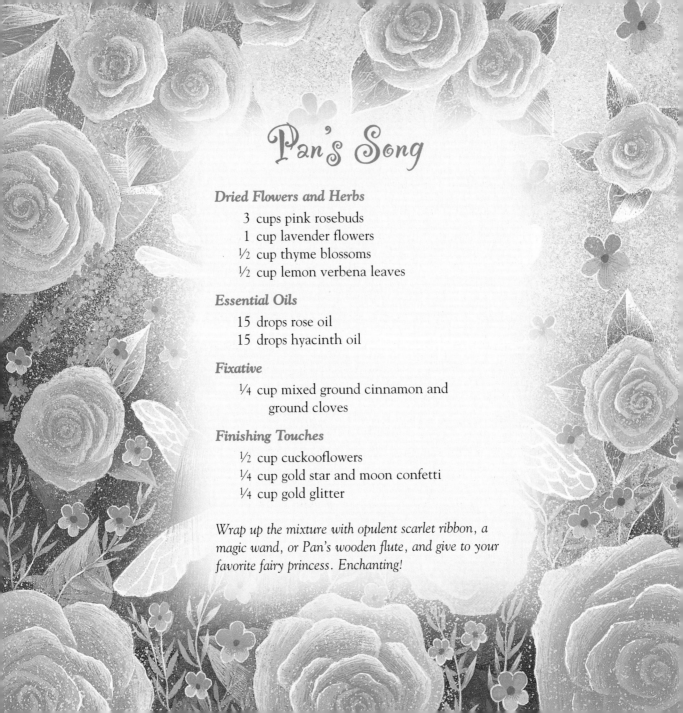

Pan's Song

Dried Flowers and Herbs

3 cups pink rosebuds
1 cup lavender flowers
½ cup thyme blossoms
½ cup lemon verbena leaves

Essential Oils

15 drops rose oil
15 drops hyacinth oil

Fixative

¼ cup mixed ground cinnamon and
ground cloves

Finishing Touches

½ cup cuckooflowers
¼ cup gold star and moon confetti
¼ cup gold glitter

Wrap up the mixture with opulent scarlet ribbon, a magic wand, or Pan's wooden flute, and give to your favorite fairy princess. Enchanting!

Cuckooflower

Such a jovial little woodland bloomer: Cuckooflower springs up in surprising places, then disappears for a year or two, only to return again in sudden, shimmering profusion!

The English country folk believed that cuckooflowers belonged to the fairies, and that you never should pick them. Taking them into the house was also bad luck. Cuckoo got its name from the European bird "who doth begin to sing when the plant begins to bloom." Other folk names for this early mustard plant include may-flower, cuckoo spit, milkmaids, and, from Shakespeare's *Love's Labour's Lost*, "lady smocks all silver white," referring to the blossoms' resemblance to a chemise.

Wild thyme

Bees, which are thought to be messengers of the gods, have a particular fondness for the fresh scent of thyme; and we know that fairies do as well. Today it is a favorite of herb gardeners, who often plant thyme in rock borders and among stone paths. On the nights when little fairy feet tread lightly upon the wild herb, we can all experience the lively fragrance of fairy magic!

Thyme grows as a ground cover, with lovely lavender blossoms, and is it is said fairies hide their babies here for safekeeping. The essential oil has an antiseptic aroma, and is used medicinally.

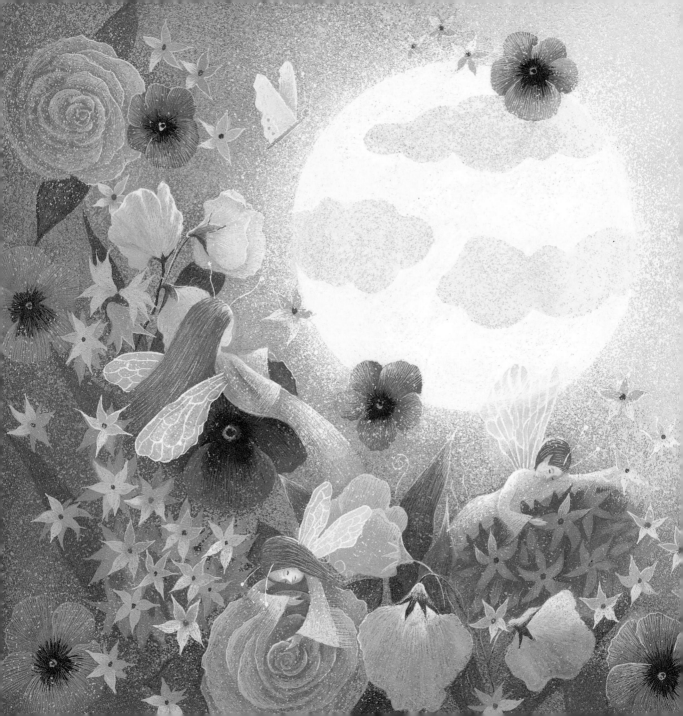

Midsummer Night's Dream

Heady red rosebuds, compelling sweet peas

and lush grape hyacinths, savory mint and soothing

lavender — these create the seductive symphony

of the garden on midsummer's eve.

The garden nymphs are silent now, resting on the

damp green carpet. They watch clouds glide across

the sky as the captive moon awaits the dawn.

This is a beautiful blend of summer's
vibrant palette of colors and scents.

Midsummer Night's Dream

Dried Flowers and Herbs

   2 cups red rosebuds
   1 cup grape hyacinth flowers
   1 cup sweet pea blossoms
  ½ cup lavender flowers
  ½ cup lemon verbena leaves
  ½ cup mint leaves

Essential Oils

 20 drops tuberose oil
  8 drops bergamot oil
  4 drops lemon verbena oil

Fixative

  ¼ cup mixed ground cinammon and
     ground cloves

Finishing Touches

  ¼ cup pressed and gilded pansy flowers
  ¼ cup blue star confetti

Wrap with a beautiful blue-violet satin ribbon. Accompanied by a box of chocolates or a bottle of good red wine, celebrate the glory of a summer night with someone you love!

Sweet pea

This dainty, beguiling summer posy is associated with a very plain young maid. One day she was visited by a fairy, disguised as an old woman, who offered her the gift of beauty if, for one year, she would do a good deed every day and never look in the mirror. When the fairy vanished, she left behind an inconspicuous little pastel plant in a pot. When the girl saw the plant, she cried, "You little darling sweet pea."

One year later the girl's face had, indeed, taken on a gentle beauty, like that of the sweet pea.

Sweet pea comes from the Latin *papilion*, meaning "butterfly," which the open blossoms resemble.

Pansy

The cheery little pansy is a flower with a heritage of fairy lore. One evening in midsummer, as the fairies were preparing their annual gala, they decided to do something to make the world brighter for the human race. They took blue from the sky, red from the sunset, yellow from a sunbeam, and brown from the earth, and worked feverishly all the night through. And that's how the glowing pansy, complete with a whimsical little face, was born.

Pansy is also associated with legends of love and with the healing of a broken heart; thus, its folk names include heartsease, love-in-idleness, tickle-my-fancy, kiss-her-in-the-pantry, and, of course, Johnny-jump-up.

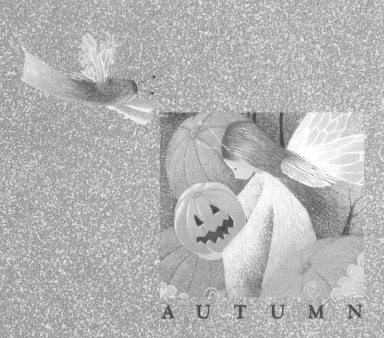

AUTUMN

Autumn Fragrances

The earthy colors and scents of the equinox

celebrate the depth of the secret presence at the

heart of nature, as autumn arrives with a vibrancy

even in its dying, so sweet and sensual.

The hillside is ablaze with burnished copper leaves,

russet vines, ripe red berries, and velvety mosses,

as this glorious season seduces the earth.

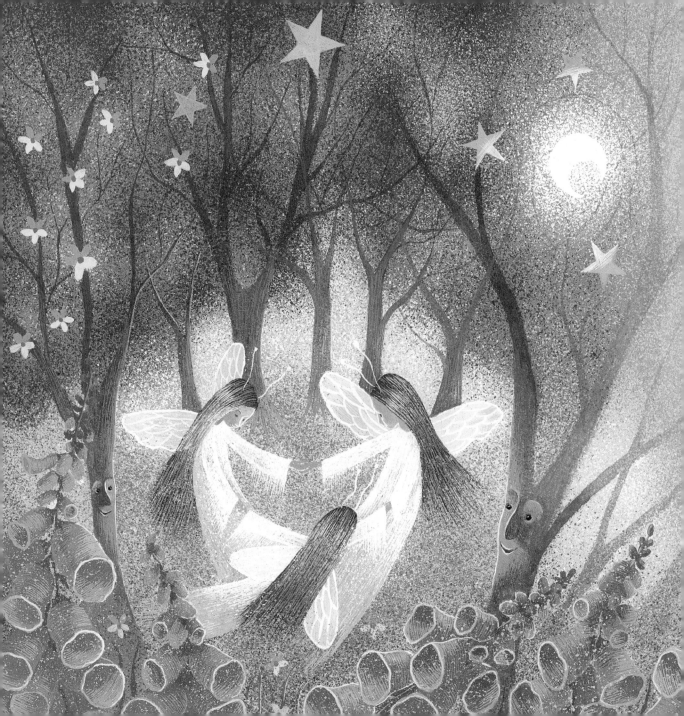

Enchanted Forest

Twilight in the forest is the most magical time of all.

The earth exhales the heat of day, and the warm air exudes

the fragrance of night. The flowers and trees glow

as though lit from within . . . stars before the stars come

out. The blue moon peeks through the evergreen sentinels,

and the fairies of the night spread their iridescent wings.

Everything sparkles like silver pennies!

Enchanted Forest is rich in balsam, vanilla, and patchouli — earthy, sensual, and mysterious. It is gorgeous in forest greens and shades of brown, with sprinkles of moonlight thrown in.

Enchanted Forest

Dried Flowers and Herbs

    2 cups deer's-tongue leaves
    2 cups patchouli leaves
    1 cup balsam fir needles

Essential Oils

    20 drops patchouli oil
    10 drops sandalwood oil
    8 drops vanilla oil

Fixative

    ¼ cup cut or ground oakmoss

Textured Elements

    ½ cup orange peel
    ½ cup sassafras root bark
    ¼ cup sandalwood chips
    ¼ cup cinnamon chips
    ¼ cup vanilla bean chunks

Finishing Touches

    ¼ cup vervain blossoms
    ¼ cup silver-painted pinecones
    ¼ cup foxglove flowers
    ¼ cup silver glitter

A very bulky blend, this makes a wonderful gift for all fairy kings. Tie it up with gobs of forest green ribbon and a gilded balsam branch. Sumptuous!

Blue vervain

Slender "blue candles" of the wild, vervain stand along meadows, pond banks, and wastelands in the heat of summer.

Vervain was first used by the ancient Druids in their lustral water and for divination and incantations. It is said that fairies and priests have used this herb to drive away evil spirits.

After the Druids introduced the herb to the Romans, it became known as an aphrodisiac and was dedicated to Venus, the goddess of love; hence the name *verbena*, which means "herb of Venus."

Vervain has many folk names: herb of grace, holy herb, herb of the cross, frog's feet, pigeon grass, and Simpler's joy.

Foxglove

It was believed that if you picked the tall spires of foxgloves — the most legendary of fairy flowers — you would offend the fairies, but growing them in your garden would surely please the pixies!

The delicate pink or white, bell-shaped blossoms are covered with tiny flecks that are said to be fairy fingerprints.

Foxglove derives its folk names of fairy gloves and fairy caps from these splendid blossoms, which became props when the fairies played dress up. Other names include fox's glew and, because of the poison found in its exquisite "cups," witch's thimble and bloody bells.

Digitalin, obtained from the blossoms of foxglove, is used to treat heart ailments.

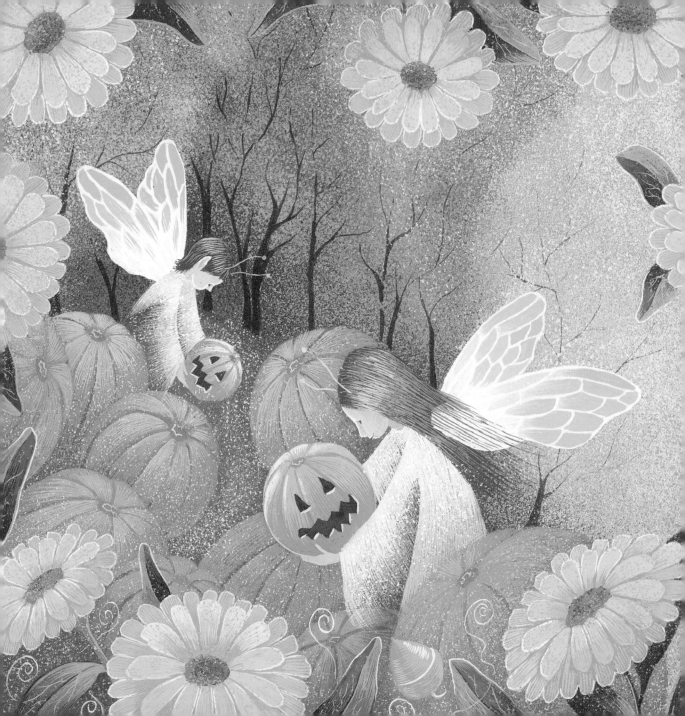

All Hallows' Eve

Beware of witches gliding across the moon,

and fat black cats! Hear the rustle of crisp maple leaves

and inhale the aroma of rich, musky earth,

spicy jack-o'-lantern, and sweet apple pie

cooling on the windowsill . . .

This is the exotic, earthy scent of All Hallows' Eve. The sandalwood, cinnamon, apple, and mint blend to create a rich and delicious fragrance.

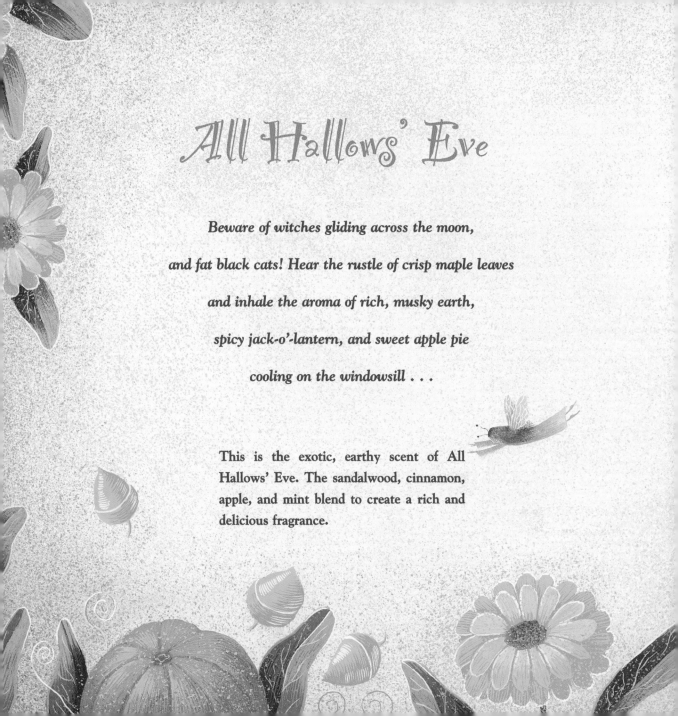

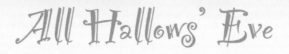

All Hallows' Eve

Dried Flowers and Herbs

    1 cup calendula flowers
    1 cup spearmint leaves

Essential Oils

    20 drops cinnamon oil
    15 drops sandalwood oil

Fixative

    ¼ cup mixed ground cinnamon and ground cloves

Textured Elements

    2 cups dried apple pieces
    ½ cup sandalwood chips
    ½ cup broken cinnamon sticks
    ¼ cup whole cloves
    ¼ cup calamus root

Finishing Touches

    ½ cup honeysuckle blossoms
    ½ cup gilded acorns
    ¼ cup toadstools
    ¼ cup black bat and silver moon confetti

Loaded with nuts, pods, berries, and spices, this blend makes the perfect hostess gift for all autumn celebrations. Fill a pumpkin shell and tie it up with a silky, honey-colored ribbon and a couple of cinnamon sticks for a festive touch. Scrumptious!

Honeysuckle

An ancient vine of waysides and tangled woodlands, honeysuckle is also known as goat's leaf and woodbine.

The lovely, caramel-colored, trumpet-shaped blossoms are intensely sweet. Bees, hummingbirds, and deer all love the delectable nectar.

Because it was often thought of as an aphrodisiac, parents forbade young girls to sleep in a room with honeysuckle: They feared it would inspire lustful dreams!

Honeysuckle was another favorite of Shakespeare's; he wrote of it in describing the fairies' revelries on midsummer's eve, when the intoxicating fragrance "lulled fairies into dancing and delight."

Toadstools

Fairy rings are often seen deep in the woodlands, surrounded by large, luminous, mysterious mushrooms. Combined with their rapid growth, toadstools have led people to believe that they belong to the fairies.

The common toadstool is in some places called pixie stool; another species of fungus is known as pixie puff. In Shakespeare's *Tempest*, we find a reference to pixie rings:

"You demi-puppets that
By moonshine do the green sour ringlets make,
Whereof the ewe not bites, and you whose
   pastime
Is to make midnight Mushrooms, that rejoice
To hear the solemn curfew."

The red fly agaric is considered the most sacred toadstool; its poisonous, hallucinogenic extracts are said to induce wicked visions and wild dancing.

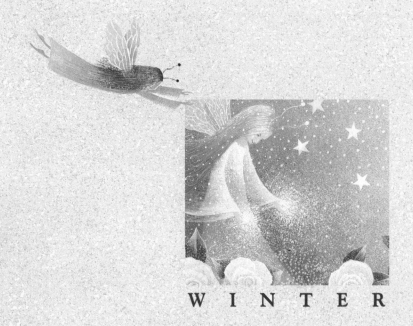

WINTER

Winter Fragrances

Forest denizens hold their breath in frosty silence

as trees, mountains, fields, and flowers

are released from the burden of exposure.

Each creature creeps back into its own nature

in the comfort of the dark, as the earth rests

and readies itself for another rebirth in the spring,

and our circular journey of life continues . . .

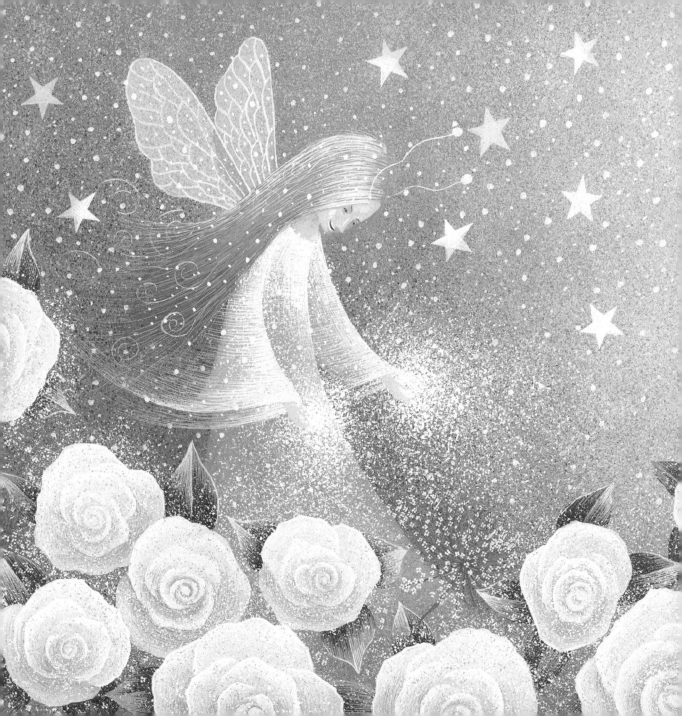

The Snow Queen

The first blush of snow covers the earth

in a cloak of glistening white,

silencing footsteps so hearts may be heard.

The Snow Queen comes tiptoeing into the still night,

casting her spell over the garden, frosting snowflakes

and icicles sweet as sugar cubes.

This is a lovely blend, brimming with linen white rosebuds and Queen-Anne's-lace, a bit of lavender, and lush winter greens. The scent is sensually sweet — rose mingled with spicy fresh bay laurel and cinnamon.

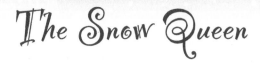

The Snow Queen

Dried Flowers and Herbs

    2 cups gilded *freshly dried* bay leaves
    2 cups white rosebuds
    1 cup lavender flowers

Essential Oils

    20 drops rose oil
    10 drops bay oil
    6 drops neroli oil

Fixative

    ¼ cup mixed ground cinnamon and ground cloves

Textured Elements

    ¼ cup whole cloves
    ½ cup cinnamon sticks (broken just a bit)

Finishing Touches

    6 pressed Queen-Anne's-lace blossoms
    ½ cup silver-painted pinecones
    ¼ cup silver glitter

Wrapped in a creamy white lace doily tied up with gauzy white ribbon, along with a book of fairy lore . . . could there be a more perfect winter gift?

Queen-Anne's-lace

This pristine white, lacy-headed wildflower with a dark center is a member of the parsley family, about which legends abound. Crowns of parsley were worn by the victors in the Grecian games. Mourners laid parsley on graves to show that their loved ones were still remembered.

The strongly scented Queen-Anne's-lace is sometimes called bee's nest, or bird's-nest root: It looks as though it is beckoning the wild critters as it dries to form a podlike enclosure.

It also was said to look like the lace doily upon which Queen Anne was knitting when she pricked her finger, causing a drop of blood to fall into the center.

Lavender

The delicate, silver-green leaves of this perennial herb form an attractive backdrop for the dense spikes of luscious purple-blue flowers. It is lavender's gentle, sweet scent — found in fresh and dried flowers as well as in its essential oil — that makes it so unforgettable and versatile.

Lavender comes from *lavare*, a Latin word meaning "to wash." According to legend, Mary washed the Christ child's clothes and hung them to dry on a lavender bush. When she went to get them, they smelled crisp and clean.

Herbalists and aromatherapists use lavender today for calming and soothing and as an antiseptic.

Christmas Magick

Christmas arrives without restraint. Holiday elves

sing songs of mayhem and magic as they deck the halls

with glitter and glitz. Seductive rose, spicy cinnamon,

sweet orange, and exhilarating pine

scent this joyful season and this succulent blend,

summoning us back to a time of wonder

and enchantment.

The green cedar tips, deep red rose hips,
and pomegranate stars are lavished with
bejeweling touches of gold.

Christmas Magick

Dried Flowers and Herbs

 2 cups gilded cedar tips
 1 cup deep red rosebuds

Essential Oils

 20 drops rose oil
 10 drops bergamot oil
 4 drops pine oil

Fixative

 ¼ cup mixed ground cinnamon and ground cloves

Textured Elements

 1 cup cinnamon chips
 ½ cup rose hips
 ½ cup juniper berries
 ½ cup cut orange rind

Finishing Touches

 6 slices dried orange
 6 slices dried pomegranate
 2 whole gilded pomegranates
 1 whole gilded orange
 12 assorted gilded pinecones
 ¼ cup periwinkle blossoms
 ¼ cup gold star confetti

A wonderfully opulent blend, Christmas Magick is the perfect companion to every holiday gift. Festoon with golden ribbons and twinkling jingle bells, or pile it high in an antique silver bowl for your holiday centerpiece.

Periwinkle

Once called the sorcerer's violet, periwinkle was thought to possess magical properties, and was used in many charms and potions. Superstition held that you should never bring fewer than seven blossoms into the house, for that would surely bring bad luck. Periwinkle was also worn in buttonholes as a protection against witches.

Also known as blue buttons, band plant, and running myrtle, this plant was thought by the Germans to bring immortality. The Belgians said that if periwinkle leaves were eaten by a man and woman together, it would create love between them. Today, the blue blossoms are a symbol of fidelity and friendship.

Rose

At the heart of the rose lies mystery and romance, a proposal of passion to come.

Legend says that Flora, goddess of flowers, overcome by the death of her favorite nymph, implored all other gods to turn her immortal essence into a mortal flower. Apollo bestowed on the rose the power of the sun, Bacchus bathed it in nectar, and Venus gave it beauty and color. Known today as the universal symbol for love — the queen of flowers — there is no equal to the incredible rose.

After Europe's "conversion" to Christianity, the rose was forbidden to be used as a symbol of the Virgin Mary because of its earlier associations with pagan deities, and lust. The purer lily was chosen as her floral symbol.

To See the Fairies

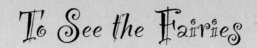

According to legend, the best times to see fairies are on the winter and summer solstices, the spring and autumn equinoxes, May Day, and Halloween. And, of course, any blue-moon summer night is also a favorable time for a sighting.

Lewis Carroll says that there are rules for sighting fairies: "First is that is must be a *very* hot day — that we may consider settled: and you must be just a *little* sleepy — but not too sleepy to keep your eyes open, mind.

"Well, and you ought to feel a little — what one may call 'fairyish' — the Scotch call it 'eerie,' and perhaps that's a prettier word; if you don't know what it means, I'm afraid I can hardly explain it; you must wait till you meet a Fairy, and then you'll know.

"And the last rule is, that the crickets should not be chirping. I can't explain that: you must take it on trust for the present.

"So, if all these things happen together, you have a good chance of seeing a Fairy — or at least a much better chance than if they didn't."

Magical Sources

ESSENTIAL OILS

Aroma Land
Route 20, Box 29AL
Santa Fe, NM 87505
(800) 938-5267

**The Essential Oil
Company**
P.O. Box 206
Lake Oswego, OR 97034
(800) 729-5912

**Frontier Cooperative
Herbs**
P.O. Box 118
Norway, IA 52318
(800) 669-3275

Herb Aromatic
25063 Oak Ridge Court
Hayward, CA 94541
(510) 886-7729

Herbal Endeavours
3618 South Emmons
Avenue
Rochester Hills, MI 48063
(810) 852-0796

Lavender Lane
7337 #1 Roseville Road
Sacramento, CA 95842
(888) 593-4400

Leydet Aromatic Oils
P.O. Box 2354
Fair Oaks, CA 95628
(916) 965-7546

Lifetree Aromatix
3949 Longridge Avenue
Sherman Oaks, CA 91423
(818) 986-0594

Oak Valley Herb Farm
P.O. Box 2482
Nevada City, CA 95959
Write for catalog.

Original Swiss Aromatics
P.O. Box 6723
San Rafael, CA 94915
(415) 459-3998

Prima Fleur Botanicals
1201-R Anderson Drive
San Rafael, CA 94901
(415) 455-0956

**Simpler Botanical
Company**
P.O. Box 39
Forestville, CA 95436
Write for catalog.

DRIED BOTANICAL
MATERIALS

Bittersweet
800 South 900 West
Etna Green, IN 46524
(219) 353-7948

Goodwin Creek Gardens
P.O. Box 83
Williams, OR 97544
(541) 846-7357

Herb Depot
124 Tecumseh Street
Dundee, MI 48131
(313) 529-3410

Lucia's Garden
2942 Virginia Street
Houston, TX 77098
(713) 523-6494

Mountain Rose Herbs
20818 High Street
North San Juan, CA
95960
(800) 879-3337

Oak Ridge Farms, Inc.
P.O. Box 28
Basking Ridge, NJ 07920
(800) 444-8843

The Rosemary House
120 S. Market Street
Mechanicsburg, PA 17055
(717) 697-5111

**San Francisco Herb
Company**
250 14th Street
San Francisco, CA 94103
(800) 227-4530

Well-Sweep Herb Farm
205 Mount Bethel Road
Port Murray, NJ 07865
(908) 852-5390

Wonderland Herbs
1305 Railroad Avenue
Bellingham, WA 98225
(360) 592-5943

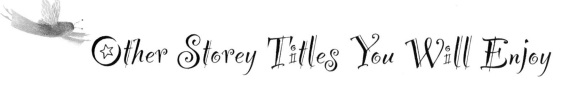

Other Storey Titles You Will Enjoy

At Home with Herbs: Inspiring Ideas for Cooking, Crafts, Decorating, and Cosmetics,
by Jane Newdick. 224 pages. Hardcover. ISBN 0-88266-886-2.

Growing Your Herb Business, by Bertha Reppert. 192 pages. Paperback.
ISBN 0-88266-612-6.

The Herbal Body Book: A Natural Approach to Healthier Hair, Skin, and Nails,
by Stephanie Tourles. 128 pages. Paperback. ISBN 0-88266-880-3.

The Herb Gardener: A Guide for All Seasons, by Susan McClure. 240 pages.
Hardcover: ISBN 0-88266-910-9. Paperback: ISBN 0-88266-873-0.

**The Herbal Home Remedy Book: Simple Recipes for Tinctures, Teas, Salves, Tonics,
and Syrups,** by Joyce A. Wardwell. 176 pages. Paperback. ISBN 1-58017-016-1.

**The Herbal Home Spa: Naturally Refreshing Wraps, Rubs, Lotions, Masks, Oils, and
Scrubs,** by Greta Breedlove. 208 pages. Paperback. ISBN 1-58107-005-6.

**Herbal Treasures: Inspiring Month-by-Month Projects for Gardening, Cooking, and
Crafts,** by Phyllis V. Shaudys. 320 pages. Paperback. ISBN 0-88266-618-5.

Making Bentwood Trellises, Arbors, Gates & Fences, by Jim Long. 144 pages.
Paperback. ISBN 1-58017-051-X.

Making Herbal Dream Pillows, by Jim Long. 64 pages. Hardcover. ISBN 1-58017-075-7.

These books and other Storey books are available at your bookstore, farm store, garden center,
or directly from Storey Books, Schoolhouse Road, Pownal, Vermont 05261,
or by calling 1-800-441-5700. Or visit our web site at www.storey.com.

Cannon, Linda.
   Creating fairy garden
fragrances.

709.1
G12

Date Due

FEB 8 1999			
MAR 0 4 1999			
MAR 2 5 1999			
NOV 2 6 1999			
NOV 1 1 2010			